The Pranayama Journal

of related interest

Restoring Prana
A Therapeutic Guide to Pranayama and Healing Through the Breath
for Yoga Therapists, Yoga Teachers, and Healthcare Practitioners
Robin L. Rothenberg
Forewords by Richard Miller and Kirsteen Wright
ISBN 978 1 84819 401 4
eISBN 978 0 85701 357 6

Svadhyaya Breath Journal
A Companion Workbook to Restoring Prana
Robin L. Rothenberg
ISBN 978 1 78775 258 0

Yoga Teaching Handbook
A Practical Guide for Yoga Teachers and Trainees
Edited by Sian O'Neill
ISBN 978 1 84819 355 0
eISBN 978 0 85701 313 2

Developing a Yoga Home Practice
An Exploration for Yoga Teachers and Trainees
Alison Leighton with Joe Taft
Edited by Sian O'Neill
ISBN 978 1 78775 704 2
eISBN 978 1 78775 705 9

The PRANAYAMA *Journal*

SINGING DRAGON

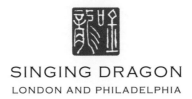

SINGING DRAGON
LONDON AND PHILADELPHIA

First published in Great Britain in 2025 by Singing Dragon, an imprint of Jessica Kingsley Publishers
Part of John Murray Press

1

Copyright © Singing Dragon 2025

 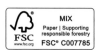
A CIP catalogue record for this title is available from the British Library and the Library of Congress

ISBN 978 1 80501 323 5
eISBN 978 1 80501 324 2

Printed and bound in Great Britain by Bell & Bain Limited

Jessica Kingsley Publishers' policy is to use papers that are natural, renewable and recyclable
products and made from wood grown in sustainable forests. The logging and manufacturing
processes are expected to conform to the environmental regulations of the country of origin.

Singing Dragon
Carmelite House
50 Victoria Embankment
London EC4Y 0DZ

www.singingdragon.com

John Murray Press
Part of Hodder & Stoughton Limited
An Hachette UK Company

FSC
www.fsc.org
MIX
Paper | Supporting
responsible forestry
FSC® C007785

Contents

❧ TECHNIQUES ❧

⚘ 28-DAY PRANAYAMA PLAN ⚘

Disclaimer

The information contained in this book is not intended to replace the services of trained medical professionals or to be a substitute for medical advice. The exercises described in this book may not be suitable for everyone to follow. You are advised to consult a doctor before embarking on any complementary therapy programme and on any matters relating to your health, and in particular on any matters that may require diagnosis or medical attention.

INTRODUCTION

❧ HOW TO USE THIS BOOK ❧

Welcome to *The Pranayama Journal*! This book is your guide to cultivating a regular *pranayama* and breathwork practice. In these pages, you'll find a selection of exercises and techniques to help you explore the powerful benefits of *pranayama* and breathwork.

The book is structured around 28 days of breathwork and *pranayama* exercises, starting with foundational techniques in the first week and building to more advanced techniques in Weeks 2, 3, and 4. As the weeks progress and you become more familiar with each practice, you might like to play with different combinations of exercises from those suggested in this journal – lean into your intuition and create the practice that feels right for you.

You can spend as little as 5 minutes on each day's practice, but feel free to spend more time repeating exercises and journalling your thoughts and observations, if you have the time. If you miss a day or two, don't panic – you can pick up where you left off on the next day. Remember that the goal is to be consistent, and consistency can take a while to develop.

Even if you're already familiar with the techniques in this book and don't consider yourself a complete beginner, it can be helpful to revisit foundational breathwork practices to refine techniques and get started with a good footing for creating a regular habit. The aim of this book is to help you to find the time and space to dedicate to *pranayama* and breathwork by starting with short and basic practices, before moving on to more complex exercises.

You can find instructions for each practice throughout the book. If you prefer to listen to the instructions, you can access audio recordings at https://library.jkp.com/redeem using the code WLDEQJK.

You might find it helpful to familiarise yourself with each practice before beginning your 28 days of *pranayama* and journalling.

You might choose to do your daily practice as soon as you wake up, or before you go to bed, or find another time to fit it into your day. We've noted where a practice is particularly energising or calming, so you can consider what time of day would be best to do these practices. What's important is finding a dedicated time for *pranayama*. Some people like to follow the habit stacking method (Mosley, 2023), where you add a new habit to an existing one, to make it easier to adopt a new routine. Could you fit in your practice before you brush your teeth, or after walking the dog, or after finishing work for the day?

If you find it tricky to make time for a regular practice, you could try scheduling 5–10 minutes each day into your calendar and setting an alarm to remind you to pick up this journal and do that day's practice. You could also agree with a friend to work through the journal together; if you aren't able to meet up to practise, you could simply agree on a time where you'll pick up this book and check in with each other once your practice is complete.

Journalling

This symbol indicates a space for you to journal your thoughts, feelings, and observations.

You are encouraged to write down your thoughts after each practice, and how you do this is up to you. There is space for you to journal in this book, or, if you prefer, you can use another notebook if you want to make longer notes. You might prefer to write in short notes or bullet points, longer paragraphs, or perhaps even sketch or draw. This is your personal guide, so don't spend time worrying about what others might think or say. Instead, think of the journalling activities as your opportunity to document your progress. You might notice big and transformational changes, or perhaps progress might be more subtle over time. There is no right or wrong approach, rather an invitation to do what feels right for you.

As part of the journalling practice, you might like to consider reflecting on: physical sensations; your emotions as you begin each practice and whether these have changed when you complete that day's practice; whether you felt focused or distracted (or somewhere in between). You might also like to note whether you have found it easy to make time for your practice, and perhaps also any challenges or barriers to cultivating a daily breathwork habit.

Keep this book with you and, ideally, in sight to remind you to pick it up for your daily practice. You might also like to use other prompts, such as setting a reminder on your phone, but hopefully over time the practices will become a natural part of your routine.

To start things off, try journalling for a few minutes about why you'd like to cultivate a regular breathwork practice.

If you're feeling stuck or unmotivated over the next 28 days, or beyond, you can revisit your notes here to remind yourself of why a breathwork practice is important to you.

Your Pranayama Toolkit

Over the next four weeks, you may also find it helpful to make a note of the practices you find particularly energising, so you can return to these at any time when you need a lift. Focus too on the practices you find calming, so you can draw on these when you're feeling anxious and want to restore balance and regulate your nervous system. Journal prompts are included throughout the book to help you with this. The practices in this book, along with the many other *pranayama* practices not included in these pages, can help you to form your own personal toolkit of practices that bring self-awareness, calmness, and vitality as you navigate the stressors of modern life.

Think of this book as a starting point that can be returned to at any time when you want to get back into the flow of a regular breathwork practice. When you feel confident doing the exercises listed in this book, we encourage you to take this self-practice further by seeking out other *pranayama* practices. You can find some suggested further reading in the Further Resources section at the end of this journal.

Precautions

Precautions (or contraindications) are included with the description of each *pranayama* exercise. You will know your own health best, and if you have any health conditions, it is important that you consult your doctor before doing the breath exercises in this journal. If something feels wrong, do not continue with that practice.

❧ WHAT IS PRANA? ❧

Prana is often referred to as our 'vital energy', or 'life force'. In ancient traditions, including yoga and Ayurveda, *prana* is the energy we need to carry out all of our basic activities. It is what sustains us and keeps us going. *Prana* can be found in the food we eat and the air we breathe, which is why *pranayama* is often associated with breathing exercises.

The Gunas and Doshas

The three *gunas* are said to be the three qualities or attributes that are present in all things. They are:

- *rajas* – relates to activeness
- *sattva* – relates to a sense of harmonious balance, peacefulness
- *tamas* – relates to inertia, sluggishness.

To exist in an ideal state, we want the *gunas* to co-exist in a balanced state. For example, not enough *tamas* and we may feel over-energised and ungrounded. *Rajas* can provide us with drive, but too much can make us feel anxious and restless. *Sattva* can be seen as a middle point between *tamas* and *rajas* and helps provide clarity and a focused mind. *Pranayama* can help to increase *sattva* by balancing *rajasic* and *tamasic* qualities.

Under the Ayurvedic system, we're all made up of the three *doshas*: *vata*, *pitta*, and *kapha*. Finding out your dominant Ayurvedic *doshic* type can also influence the best *pranayama* techniques for you. It is recommended to consult an Ayurvedic doctor to find out your *doshic* type. We could write a whole book on the *doshas*, and in fact there are many excellent resources already available, so we have included some suggested reading in the Further Resources section on page 136 if you would like to learn more.

To maintain a state of balance and feel our best selves, we need to nurture our *prana* and be conscious of how we cultivate it. With care and attention to *prana* we can flourish and feel strong, but if we neglect it, we may feel tired and unbalanced. *Prana* flows through our *nadis* (channels or pathways). When these channels are blocked, *prana* becomes stuck, disrupting the delicate balance in the body. A regular *pranayama* practice helps us to cultivate our vital energy and keep our *nadis* clear of blockages.

Think also of the five *koshas* or layers of the self – our *pranamaya kosha* (energetic layer) sits between our *annamaya kosha* (physical layer) and *manomaya kosha* (mental layer). *Prana* is the connection between body and mind, so by bringing awareness to this layer through breathwork and *pranayama* practices, we work on harnessing our vitality for optimal wellbeing.

❧ NOTES ON SITTING/LYING DOWN ☙

For most of the *pranayama* exercises we give in the journal, you'll often find that we recommend being seated for the duration of the practice. Most of us will not be used to sitting upright for extended periods of time unless you have a regular yoga or meditation practice. Even if you're a seasoned yogi, we wanted to dedicate time to give you some pointers on how to sit comfortably and maintain an upright posture. There are several reasons why paying attention to how you sit for your *pranayama* practice is useful. Here are just a few:

- Sitting comfortably means that you're less likely to get distracted during your practice. Feeling the need to fidget and constantly readjust your position means that you lose focus on your breath.

- Maintaining an upright spine where you aren't slumping forward and rounding the shoulders is better for your back and shoulders and will improve your posture.

- Having a comfortable upright posture will allow you to breathe more freely as you're giving the lungs space to expand and contract without restrictions.

For some of us, sitting on the floor is just not comfortable for several minutes at a time. If this sounds like you, consider sitting on a chair (ideally something adjustable) that supports your back and allows you to place your feet flat on the floor. Your knees should be directly above the ankles and your thighs parallel to the floor (if the knees are higher than the hips, consider adjusting the height of the chair or sitting on a cushion; if the knees are lower than the hips, consider adjusting the height of the chair or placing a cushion or folded blanket beneath your feet).

If you're sitting on the floor but find yourself regularly slumping forward and rounding the upper back and shoulders, you could try sitting with your back against a wall. Your spine will still maintain its natural curves, but having the physical reminder of the wall may help you to stay upright for longer. After a few sessions, you can experiment with sitting away from the wall to see if this has helped you to habitually sit up taller.

Sitting in *sukhasana* (cross-legged) is a common position in which to practise breathwork. You may feel very comfortable here, but here are some tips to help you maintain a comfortable seat:

- If you find that your knees are higher than your hips when sitting cross-legged, try sitting on something to elevate your seat. This could be one or several yoga blocks, a meditation cushion, or something else. This will allow the knees to drop down and let the hips feel more open.

- You may notice that you get pins and needles in your feet and/or ankles when sitting cross-legged for more than a couple of minutes. If this sounds like you, you could place a folded blanket underneath the feet to cushion them.

- Likewise, it can feel comfortable to place a rolled-up blanket or a couple of cushions between the outer shins and inner ankles, which takes the pressure off the ankles and allows the knees and hips to relax.

Some other seated options for practising *pranayama* are:

- Kneeling, either sitting on the heels or on one or more yoga blocks. If you feel pressure on the knees while kneeling, you can try placing a rolled-up blanket or towel behind the backs of the knees, which reduces the bend in the knees.

- Lotus pose, where you sit cross-legged with both feet placed on the opposite thigh. To sit in this position comfortably and safely, you'll need to have very open hips and knees. Do not force yourself into lotus or half-lotus pose as this may risk injury.

- Sitting on a meditation stool. A meditation stool is a great option for anyone that finds sitting for long periods uncomfortable as it elevates your seat and takes the pressure off the feet and ankles.

Another option for some practices is to lie down. Ideally, this would be flat on the floor, using either a yoga mat or blanket underneath you. If this isn't possible due to space constraints, you could lie down on your bed, but you may end up falling asleep, especially for some of the more relaxing *pranayama* practices!

Here are some tips for setting yourself up for a reclined *pranayama* practice:

- Lying flat on your back with the legs stretched out, feet relaxed, and your arms by your side with the palms of the hands facing up is a great starting point. This is often called *savasana* or corpse pose.

- If you have any niggles in the lower back, you may find it more comfortable to bend your knees and place your feet flat on the floor at least hip width apart. Here, you can allow the knees to rotate inwards so that the inner knees touch in the centre.

- You may find it comfortable to place a blanket, cushion, or yoga block behind the head for support. The aim is to keep the chin roughly parallel with the rest of your face. If the chin is lifted, you may need to prop the head more, and if you feel like the chin is tucked too close to the chest, you may need to lessen the height of any props behind the head.

- If you find that lying still is uncomfortable because the floor is too hard, consider adding additional padding, such as an additional yoga mat or extra blanket(s).

- Similarly, if you feel cold when lying still, cover yourself with a blanket or add extra layers of clothing. Your body temperature is likely to drop when lying still for several minutes.

- In many yoga classes, especially yin or restorative classes, students are offered the option to use sandbags and weighted props to help the body relax deeply. We won't go into great detail about this here, as we assume that not everyone has access to these props, but if you're used to practising with sandbags, etc., please feel free to experiment here, always being mindful that any sandbags or weighted blankets should not restrict your breathing in any way.

☙ A NOTE ON NASAL BREATHING ❧

For many of the practices in this journal, we recommend that you breathe in and out of the nose. Of course, if you have any restrictions to breathing through the nose, such as a cough or cold or allergies, then just breathe comfortably. However, there are myriad benefits to nasal breathing!

Breathing through your nose rather than through your mouth can help filter out things like dust and allergens and humidify the air you breathe into the lungs. Inside your nose, there are lots of tiny nasal hairs that trap things like pollen and dust so that they don't make their way further into your nasal passage. The anatomy of your nose helps the incoming air slow down to enable it to warm up and humidify before making its way into your lungs. Take a moment to breathe in and out through your nose – you might start to notice that the air coming in feels slightly cooler than the air you're breathing out. If someone tends to breathe through their mouth instead of their nose, then they may notice dryness in the mouth and increased allergies.

There is increasing evidence that nasal breathing throughout the day (and night) has many health benefits, including better sleep, reduced anxiety, increased oxygen uptake, and fewer allergies (Nestor, 2020). Therefore, practising *pranayama* techniques where the mouth remains closed is a great way to get used to nasal breathing and perhaps to breathe more consciously during your whole day.

✤ A NOTE ON THE TEXT ✤

Where applicable, we have provided the Sanskrit name for a practice in italics followed in brackets by the English transliteration or other names a practice is known by. Please also see the Glossary on pages 137–8.

Techniques

Remember, you can access audio recordings of all of the *pranayama* techniques at https://library.jkp.com/redeem using the code WLDEQJK.

You may find it easier to practise the techniques alongside the recordings at first, then eventually start to practise on your own.

FOUNDATIONAL TECHNIQUES

In this section, we will outline some foundational or beginner's *pranayama* and breathwork practices. Even if you're already familiar with the practices in this section, we encourage you to approach these practices with openness and curiosity.

Breath Awareness

Before we start our *pranayama* journey, it's useful to take a moment to tune into an awareness of the breath. If you've been practising breathwork or yoga for a while, you may be used to doing this, but it can be helpful to go back to basics!

Taking the time to notice the breath and its effects on your body and emotional and energetic states can be an incredibly effective tool to calm the nervous system and tap into the present moment. We recommend practising breath awareness at the start and end of your daily *pranayama* practice as a way of checking in to see how the various practices have affected you. It can also be used as a standalone practice.

PRECAUTIONS

* None.

BENEFITS

* Calms the nervous system.

* Focuses the mind on the present.

✳   A very simple technique that can act as a reset.

✳   Balances *prana* (energy) in the body.

PRACTICE

1. Breath awareness can be practised lying down or seated, so get into a comfortable position that you can stay in for a few minutes.

2. If you feel comfortable, close your eyes or soften your gaze and allow your eyelids to feel heavy.

3. Breathe naturally, trying not to manipulate the breath or control it in any way.

4. Once you're settled into a natural breath, take a moment to notice whether you're breathing in and out through the mouth or nose. Perhaps you're breathing in through the nose and out through the mouth, or vice versa. Or maybe you're breathing in and out through the nose, or just through the mouth. Don't try to change anything; just notice what comes naturally.

5. Now begin to pay attention to where the breath enters and leaves your body, either through the nose or mouth. Does the temperature of the air coming in feel cooler or warmer going out?

6. Take some time to be curious about the quality of your breathing. Is it fast or slow? Is the inhalation longer or shorter than the exhalation? Does the breath feel smooth and comfortable, or does it feel restricted in any way? Is it more comfortable to breathe in or breathe out, or perhaps you find both feel the same?

7. Then, when you're ready, start to bring your awareness to where you feel the physical effects of the breath in the body. You might feel movements or sensations in your throat, nasal passage, shoulders,

chest, ribs, or belly. You might even feel something in your hands or feet. Take your time here to notice your unique experience of the breath.

Next, begin to notice how your breathing makes you feel energetically or emotionally. Do you feel calm and comfortable, or do you feel anxious or stressed? Or perhaps you're somewhere in between, or you aren't quite sure. There is no right answer; just go with what comes up.

If at any point, your thoughts start to intrude on your breath awareness practice, go back to one of the earlier steps. It is perfectly normal for our minds to start thinking about something else during practice.

10. To conclude the practice, bring your focus back to your natural breath and make a mental note as to whether you notice anything different.

JOURNALLING PROMPTS

* What did you notice about your breath at the start of your practice today? Were you naturally breathing through the nose or the mouth? Was your breath fast or slow? Calm or laboured?

* How easy did you find it to maintain a focus on your breathing? Did you get easily distracted, or was it easy once you got started?

* How did you feel at the end of the practice? Were there any differences in your breathing compared to the start of the practice?

Foundational Techniques **25**

Sama Vritti (Equal Breathing): Beginner's Version

PRECAUTIONS

*   If you have low blood pressure, do not hold the breath after the exhale.

*   If you have unmedicated high blood pressure, or eye, lung, or heart problems, do not hold the breath after the inhale.

BENEFITS

*   Calms the mind and the nervous system.

*   Balances *prana* (energy) in the body.

*   Focuses the mind on the present.

*   Can help to increase lung capacity.

Sama vritti breathing is a foundational *pranayama* technique. Roughly translated from Sanskrit, *sama* means same or equal and *vritti* means fluctuations, so *sama vritti* is often referred to as equal breathing. When practising *sama vritti*, you're trying to breathe in and out for equal amounts of time, sometimes adding a breath retention after the inhalation and another retention after the exhalation.

This is an excellent technique with which to begin your breathwork journey as you can easily adjust the practice to suit you. For example, you can start by breathing in for a count of two and breathing out for a count of two, then, if you feel comfortable, you could try counting in and out for longer (always keeping the counts equal). As you repeat the practice, you may find that you can increase the length of your breaths as the weeks go by, or on some days you might prefer to keep the breaths shorter.

You might also find that your breaths start to slow down as you practice *sama vritti* regularly.

Counting the breath is also a great tool to focus your mind on the present moment; if you lose your count, you can simply start over.

PRACTICE

1. *Sama vritti* can be practised lying down or seated, so get into a comfortable position that you can stay in for a few minutes.

2. If you feel comfortable, close your eyes or soften your gaze and let your eyelids feel heavy.

3. Take a moment to breathe normally and notice how you feel in body and mind.

4. After a few breaths, start to breathe in and out through your nose (if you have a cold or any nasal restrictions, breathe in whatever way feels most comfortable).

5. When you're ready, start to count the breath, inhaling for two counts and exhaling for two counts.

6. If there are no contraindications, see if you can notice the slight pause at the end of the inhalation and the slight pause at the end of the exhalation.

7. Continue to breathe in this way for a few breaths, taking time to observe the effects of the practice.

8. If you feel ready, you can adjust the count to three or four, making sure to keep the breath equal. If the increased count is too much, you can go back to breathing in and out for two counts.

9. When you're ready to conclude the practice, stop counting and return to your natural breath, taking some time to notice the after-effects of the *pranayama practice.*

JOURNALLING PROMPTS

✳   How did you find today's practice? Was it easy to breathe in and out for equal counts?

✳   If this was challenging, what part of the breath did you find trickier, the inhalation or the exhalation?

✳   Did you try adjusting the counts, and, if so, how did that go?

✳   How did you feel at the end of the practice?

✳   Is there anything you would like to do differently next time?

Simhasana Pranayama (Lion's Breath)

PRECAUTIONS

* If you have unmedicated high blood pressure, modify the intensity of the exhalation.

* If you're experiencing eye strain, do not open your eyes too widely when exhaling.

* If you're uncomfortable in the traditional seated posture for this pose, try sitting in *sukhasana* (cross-legged) instead.

BENEFITS

* Reduces tension, especially in the head and jaw area.

* Reduces stress.

* Strengthens the muscles in your face and throat.

* Can improve lung capacity.

* Promotes better sleep.

* Balances *prana* in the body.

* Stimulates the thyroid gland.

Lion's breath is so-called because the sound when you exhale can be likened to a lion's roar. On the breath out, you should try to open your eyes and mouth as wide as you can, while sticking your tongue out and down towards your chin, making a 'hahhh' sound. You may feel a bit silly at first, but this is an excellent practice for relieving stress!

We've advised you to practise lion's breath while seated, but this breath can be incorporated into your yoga *asana* practice, for example, in postures such as *utkata konasana* (goddess pose) or *malasana* (garland pose/squat). If the kneeling posture isn't comfortable, feel free to sit in *sukhasana* (cross-legged).

PRACTICE

1. Lion's breath is best practised while seated, so either come to a comfortable seated position or sit kneeling with the knees wide and the big toes touching.

2. Take a moment to become aware of your breath, taking a few comfortable, nourishing breaths to settle your body and mind.

3. Open your eyes and breathe in through the nose.

4. If you're kneeling, place your hands in front of you with the palms facing down, fingertips pointed towards you (the wrists are facing forwards).

5. Open your eyes wide with your gaze focused on the point between your eyebrows (this is also known as *ajna chakra,* the third eye point). If you're kneeling, lean forwards on the exhale, keeping the back straight. However, if you're sitting, exhale through the mouth, sticking your tongue out as far as you can. As you exhale, make a 'hahhh' sound, a bit like a lion's roar.

6. Repeat twice more.

7. Come back to your natural breath, taking a moment to notice the effects of the practice. You can repeat this practice if you wish.

Variations note: Once you have practised this technique a few times, you can experiment with it in various yoga poses, such as *utkata konasana* (goddess pose), or *marjaryasana/bitilasana* (cat/cow pose).

JOURNALLING PROMPTS

* What was your experience physically and emotionally when practising this *pranayama* technique?

* Would you try this practice again? If so, would you adjust it in any way (e.g. more or fewer repetitions; at the end or start of your practice; at a different time of day)?

* How did it feel to use the sound of your breath in your practice?

Ujjayi Breath

(Victorious Breath/Ocean Breath): Beginner's Version

PRECAUTIONS

* Pregnancy.

* Chronic fatigue.

* Low blood pressure.

* Hypertension.

* Heart conditions.

BENEFITS

* Slows down the breath.

* Helps to calm the nervous system.

* Builds *agni* (inner fire) within the body.

* Increases energy.

* Stimulates the *vishuddha chakra* (throat chakra).

* Enhances mental focus.

Ujjayi breath is a very common *pranayama* technique used during yoga *asana* practice. However, it can be practised on its own, without holding various yoga poses, and can be a great addition to your *pranayama* toolkit.

We've included two versions of *ujjayi* in this journal, one for beginners and one for more advanced practitioners, so start with this version and, once you feel comfortable, you can try the more advanced practice.

Ujjayi is made up of two Sanskrit words – *ud* (upwards) + *jaya* (victory or success) – and is therefore translated to mean *to lift upwards* or *the breath of victory*. As well as being known as victorious breath or conqueror's breath, it's also known as ocean breath due to the soft, wave-like sound that is made by the constriction of the throat. A number of people nickname *ujjayi* as Darth Vader breath because of this, and practitioners are often encouraged to raise the volume to emphasise the sound. You can certainly experiment with this in your daily practice, but we would encourage you not to force your breath; a soft sound that only you can hear is perfectly fine.

PRACTICE

Note: Ujjayi is commonly practised when carrying out yoga *asana,* but for the purposes of this journal, we suggest you practise in stillness, at least to begin with.

1. *Ujjayi* can be practised seated or lying down, so find a comfortable position that you can stay in for a few minutes.

2. Close your eyes to avoid distractions and take a moment to tune into your natural breath, noting how it feels today, in this moment.

3. Breathe in through the nose.

4. As you breathe out, open your mouth and make a soft, slow 'haa' sound. To make this sound, you'll naturally restrict the throat. If you aren't sure if you're getting this quite right, imagine you're holding a small mirror in front of your mouth and your breath out is fogging up the mirror.

5. Once you're comfortable with this, try to breathe out with your mouth closed, still restricting the throat.

6. You should notice a soft sound, a bit like the waves of the ocean.

7. Continue to breathe with your mouth closed, restricting the throat on the exhalation.

8. When you are ready to complete the practice of *ujjayi*, release the restriction of the throat and breathe naturally, taking a moment to notice any changes to how you feel.

JOURNALLING PROMPTS

* Is this *pranayama* technique new to you or something you have tried in the past? If you have done this before, did the experience feel any different? How so?

* Did you notice any changes in the length of your exhalation once you started to use the throat to create the *ujjayi* breath? Did you notice anything else?

* Did you find it comfortable to breathe in this way? If not, what were the challenges?

* How focused did you feel in your practice today? If it's helpful, you can give yourself a score out of 10, 10 being very focused and 1 finding it very difficult to maintain your focus on your breathwork practice. Try not to get competitive or feel frustrated if you have some days when your focus was not as forthcoming. Just observe these frustrations and know that you can try again later.

Extended Exhalation

PRECAUTIONS

∗ Not suitable for anyone with severe cardiac issues or severe hypertension.

BENEFITS

∗ Promotes relaxation.

∗ Calms the nervous system.

∗ Activates the parasympathetic nervous system.

Extending the exhalation is scientifically proven to calm the nervous system, making it an excellent addition to your *pranayama* practice. Breathing in this way can stimulate the vagus nerve (also known as the 'wandering nerve'), which is part of the parasympathetic nervous system (PNS) (De Couck, *et al.,* 2019). The PNS is responsible for the 'rest and digest' response in the body, which is activated when we're feeling calm and safe.

When we're stressed or anxious, our sympathetic nervous system (SNS) activates, which switches on our body's 'fight or flight' response. When this happens, our heart rate increases, as does the speed of our breath, while blood flow increases to our skeletal muscles and decreases to our gastrointestinal system and skin. This reaction from our nervous system originates from the time when humans were hunter-gatherers and needed to escape from predators. The good news is that humans living today do not often need to escape from predators; however, the fast-paced nature of modern life, with its constant stressors, means our stress response is activated far too often. As a result, many of us are in a near-constant state of sympathetic arousal, which can affect all of the systems in our body, such as our digestion, as well as our emotional state.

When the SNS is activated due to anxiety, overwork, or stress, we can use our *pranayama* practice to stimulate the vagus and switch on the PNS to bring our body back to a state of balance (also called homeostasis). Breathing in this way sends signals to the brain that we're calm and safe.

There is evidence that breathing deeply with extended exhalations for just a couple of minutes will start to stimulate the vagus nerve and help you to feel calmer. Therefore, we recommend this practice for anyone who is feeling busy, stressed, or anxious. You might even find it useful to journal about how you're feeling before and after this practice to see if it makes any difference.

PRACTICE

1. This practice can be done seated or lying down, so make yourself comfortable and find a position to sit or lie in where you can stay for a few minutes.

2. Close your eyes or soften your gaze.

3. Take a few moments to notice your natural breath and ask yourself how you're feeling today, in this precise moment.

4. If possible, begin to breathe in and out through the nose if you're not already.

5. When you're ready, start to count the breath, breathing in for a count of two and out for a count of two.

6. Take a few even, equal breaths and, when you're ready, you can start to extend the exhalation, breathing in for two and breathing out for three or even four counts.

7. Continue to breathe in this way for at least 2 minutes if you can.

You can even make the exhalation longer if you wish. The breath should not feel forced or uncomfortable in any way.

8. When you're ready to conclude the practice, come back to your natural breath and cease counting.

9. Take a moment to note how you feel in both body and mind.

10. This practice can be repeated at any point during your day.

JOURNALLING PROMPTS

* How did you feel at the start of this practice? How did you feel by the end of this practice?

* Did anything unexpected come up for you during this practice? If so, observe how this makes you feel without judgement.

* Are there times in your life when this practice might be particularly useful? If so, remember that this practice is part of your toolkit and that you can return to it at any time.

❧ ENERGY CHANNELS ❧

In yoga theory, we're taught that the *nadis* (main energy channels) end in the nose, so the practices described here are often related to these channels. The *pingala nadi* ends in the right nostril, the *ida nadi* ends in the left nostril, and the *sushumna nadi,* which is the main channel of energy through the centre of the body, ends in the centre of the nostrils where the septum and upper lip meet. Therefore, *pingala nadi,* which is associated with more masculine, active energy, is dominant when we breathe predominantly through the right nostril and *ida nadi,* which is associated with feminine, creative, and calm energy, is more active when we breathe through the left nostril. When we breathe equally through both nostrils, *sushumna nadi* is activated, and it's thought that this leads us to feel balanced both physically and mentally.

Practices that work with the *pingala, ida,* and *sushumna nadis* are described below.

Surya Bhedana and Chandra Bhedana

(Sun-Piercing Breath and Moon-Piercing Breath)

PRECAUTIONS

* Do not practise if you're experiencing a chronic respiratory condition.

BENEFITS

* Brings calm and balance to body and mind.

* Enables becoming more mindful of the present moment.

* Increases focus and concentration.

* Lowers the heart rate.

* Balances the left and right side of the body and brain.

* Said to purify the *nadis* (the energy channels in the body) so that energy flows more freely.

* May help to remove blockages in the nose or sinuses.

Together, *surya bhedana* (sun-piercing breath) and *chandra bhedana* (moon-piercing breath) are known as alternate nostril breathing. This breathing technique is commonly used as part of a yoga practice but can easily be a standalone practice. There are several variations of alternate nostril breathing, so we'll give you a couple of options here and another later in the book.

The first practice is called *surya bhedana,* which is often translated to mean sun-piercing breath. This is traditionally seen as an energising

Foundational Techniques **41**

breath, so is practised in the morning or when you need a pick-me-up. The second practice is called *chandra bhedana,* or moon-piercing breath, and is seen as a calming practice that is traditionally done in the evening. The main difference between these practices is that *surya bhedana* begins by inhaling through the right nostril and *chandra bhedana* begins by inhaling through the left nostril.

At the start of each practice, we ask you to pay attention to your nostrils and notice whether you tend to breathe through one side of the nose or the other. It is thought that we naturally tend to breathe through one nostril for around 90 minutes and then switch to the other side (Sovik, n.d.), alternating throughout the day. This is called the nasal cycle.

If for any reason you're unable to block the nostrils with the finger/ thumb, it is also possible to visualise the air coming in and out through the nostrils, but this may take some practice.

Surya Bhedana

(Alternate Nostril Breathing/Sun-Piercing Breath)

Note: To be practised during the day, or when you need an energising practice.

1. This technique is usually practised while seated, so find a comfortable sitting position where you can sit upright comfortably for a few minutes.

2. Take a moment to breathe comfortably and begin to pay attention to your nostrils. Is one side of your nose easier to breathe through than the other, or is it difficult to tell the difference?

3. Bring your right hand in front of your face, placing your thumb on your right nostril and your ring and little fingers on the left nostril. The middle two fingers can rest in between your eyebrows, or you can tuck them in towards the palm. The left hand can rest on your lap or on your left thigh or knee.

4. Keeping the left nostril blocked, release the right nostril and breathe in.

5. Block the right nostril with the thumb, release the left nostril and breathe out.

6. Repeat, breathing in through the right nostril and out through the left nostril.

7. When you're ready to conclude the practice, release your hand and take a few breaths through both nostrils. Think back to the observations you made in step 2 and notice whether there has been any change.

JOURNALLING PROMPTS

∗ What time of day is it? How do you usually feel at this time, without having done this practice?

∗ Now that you have done this practice, what changes do you notice in yourself? It's ok if you don't feel more energised after the first attempt; you can simply try again later.

∗ How comfortable was your breath during this practice?

Chandra Bhedana

(Alternate Nostril Breathing/Moon-Piercing Breath)

Note: To be practised in the evening, or when you need a calming practice.

1. This technique is usually practised while seated, so find a comfortable sitting position where you can sit upright comfortably for a few minutes.

2. Take a moment to breathe comfortably and begin to pay attention to your nostrils. Is one side easier to breathe through than the other, or is it difficult to tell the difference?

3. Bring your right hand in front of your face, placing your thumb on your right nostril and your ring and little fingers on the left nostril. The middle two fingers can rest in between your eyebrows, or you can tuck them in towards the palm. The left hand can rest on your lap or on your left thigh or knee.

4. Keeping the right nostril blocked, release the left nostril and breathe in.

5. Block the left nostril with the thumb, release the right nostril and breathe out.

6. Repeat, breathing in through the left nostril and out through the right nostril.

7. When you're ready to conclude the practice, release your hand and take a few breaths through both nostrils. Think back to the observations you made in step 2 and notice whether there has been any change.

JOURNALLING PROMPTS

✷   What time of day is it? How do you usually feel at this time, without having done this practice?

✷   Now that you have done this practice, what changes do you notice in yourself? It's ok if you don't feel calmer after the first attempt; you can simply try again later.

✷   How comfortable was your breath during this practice? How does it compare to sun-piercing breath?

Sitali Pranayama (Cooling Breath)

PRECAUTIONS

* Because this practice cools the body, it may be best not to undertake it if you're already feeling cold or during colder months when the air is already very cool and dry as it may aggravate the lungs.

BENEFITS

* Cools the body.

* Calms the nervous system.

* Reduces fatigue.

* Reduces bad breath.

* Lowers high blood pressure.

Sitali pranayama, also known as cooling breath, is a simple practice that can help to bring down the temperature in the body and calm the nervous system. It is best practised in the summer months or if you feel an excess of heat in the body. You will see that we ask you to curl your tongue for the inhalation in this *pranayama* technique, but if that isn't possible for you (for some people, curling their tongue is out of the question!) then you can purse the lips as if you're breathing through a straw and you'll achieve the same effect.

PRACTICE

1. This *pranayama* technique is usually practised while seated, so find a comfortable sitting position that you can stay in for a few minutes.

2. Close your eyes or allow your eyelids to soften.

3. Take a few comfortable breaths and check in with your natural breath and note how you're feeling.

4. Take some time to notice the length of your inhalation and exhalation. No need to force anything, just breathe naturally.

5. Notice the temperature of the air around you and pay particular attention to the temperature of the air you're breathing in and breathing out. Is the air you breathe out warmer or cooler than the air that you're breathing in? Is the temperature the same? There's no right or wrong answer here; we're simply observing.

6. When you're ready, purse your lips and roll your tongue before taking a long, slow breath in.

7. Close your mouth and exhale through your nose.

8. Repeat for a couple of minutes, noting how the pursed lips of the inhalation might affect the temperature of the air you breathe in, the length of the inhalation and exhalation, and any other observations.

9. When you're ready to conclude the practice, come back to your regular breathing, taking time to note whether it has had any effect on you, either physically or emotionally.

JOURNALLING PROMPTS

* What effect did this cooling breath have on the rest of your body?

* Do you notice any emotional impact?

* Is there any change to your natural breathing pattern after you have completed this practice?

Bhramari Pranayama (Bee Breath)

PRECAUTIONS

* Do not practise *Bhramari pranayama* if you have an ear infection or high blood pressure.

BENEFITS

* Lowers blood pressure.

* Relieves tension, especially around the head.

* Increases the production of nitric oxide, which supports better oxygenation of the cells and tissues.

* Calms the nervous system.

* Supports dealing with anger.

* Improves focus and concentration.

The word *Bhramari* is the name of a Hindu goddess of bees. When practising this *pranayama* technique, you'll hum, making a sound like a buzzing bee, hence why this technique is called *Bhramari!* The humming sound can be as loud or as quiet as you like, but you could experiment with the volume of the humming sound as you practise this on different days to see what you prefer and what feels most comfortable. Volume and pitch have energetic effects. Loud volume and high pitch tend to be more energising, while low volume and low pitch tend to be more calming.

We have included instructions below for you to practise *Bhramari* with the traditional hand position, where the fingers block the ears and nose and keep the eyes closed. The reasoning here is that the senses of sound, sight, and smell are restricted so that your focus is primarily on the breath.

However, if you aren't comfortable with this, or you simply prefer not to use the hand position, you can place your hands in your lap, take a *mudra* (hand position) or just block the ears. Blocking the ears will make the humming sound seem much louder.

PRACTICE

1. *Bhramari pranayama* should be practised while seated, so find a comfortable sitting position where you can stay for a few minutes.

2. Close your eyes or soften your gaze.

3. Take a few comfortable, natural breaths, noticing how your breath is feeling in the present moment and how you're feeling both physically and emotionally.

4. If you would like, bring both of your hands in front of your face and spread the fingers.

5. Your thumbs should gently block your ears, your index fingers lightly touch the inner corners of your eyes, your middle fingers press against your nostrils, and your ring and little fingers press just above the upper lip and just below the bottom lip, respectively, to close your mouth.

6. Release the nostrils slightly to allow you to take an inhalation.

7. Block the nostrils and make a soft humming sound like a bee for the whole exhalation.

8. Repeat the humming breath several times. You can continue this *pranayama* technique for several minutes (between 10 and 15 minutes is fine).

9. When you're ready to conclude the practice, release your hands and

rest them in your lap. Breathe normally with your eyes still closed, noticing if the *Bhramari pranayama* has had any effects on you.

JOURNALLING PROMPTS

✳ Did you experiment with different humming pitches? Did a lower pitch have a different effect from a higher pitch?

✳ Did you experiment with different humming volumes? Did a louder humming sound have a different effect from a quieter sound?

✳ How comfortable did you find this practice? If you found it uncomfortable is there anything that you would change (maybe starting with fewer repetitions and building from there)?

✳ Are there times in your life when you need a calming practice? Would this be a good breath to keep in your toolkit?

ADVANCED TECHNIQUES

Sama Vritti

(Box Breathing/Equal Breathing): Advanced Version

PRECAUTIONS

* If you have low blood pressure, do not hold the breath after the exhalation.

* If you have high blood pressure, or eye, lung, or heart problems, do not hold the breath after the inhale.

BENEFITS

* Calms the mind and the nervous system.

* Balances *prana* (energy) in the body.

* Focuses the mind on the present.

* Can help to increase lung capacity.

* A very simple technique that can act as a reset.

Box breathing, also known as coherent breathing, is the next step on from *sama vritti pranayama,* which we covered in the foundational techniques. When practising box breathing, the aim is for all parts of the breath (the inhalation, breath retention, exhalation, and breath suspension) to be equal, just as the four sides of a box are (see image 1). You can even imagine the four sides of a box when you're practising this technique and visualise the breath travelling around each side of it.

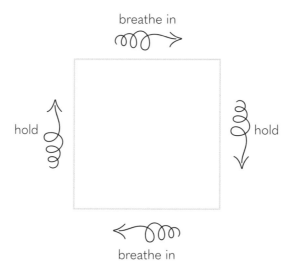

breathe in

hold

hold

breathe in

Image 1: One way to help you focus on your *sama vritti pranayama* is to visualise the four sides of a box as you breathe

This technique is proven to be extremely useful for calming the nervous system and dealing with stress. It is said that the Navy SEALS are trained in using this practice to help them deal with stress (Divine, 2016).

As with *sama vritti* (equal breathing), you can begin by breathing in for a count of two, holding for two, breathing out for a count of two, and holding the breath out for two counts. You can then build up to a longer duration, as long as you ensure all parts of the breath are equal in duration. As you repeat the practice over several weeks, you may find that you can increase the length of your breaths, or on some days you might prefer to keep the breaths shorter. You might also find that your natural breathing pattern becomes slower as you practise box breathing regularly.

The pauses between the inhalation and exhalation and vice versa are an interesting part of this particular *pranayama* technique and worth paying attention to when you practise. The retentions as you hold the breath in or out are called *kumbhaka*, which literally translates as *pot* (i.e. imagine the lungs are a pot that holds the air that you're holding in after inhale and holding out after exhale) and these pauses are described by BKS Iyengar as a 'state where there is no inhalation or exhalation' (Iyengar, 2001, p. 22). It is said that this pause leads to a stillness in the mind. When you practise breath holds, take a moment to notice how you feel in these moments when there is an absence of the breath and whether you feel the need to rush ahead into the next breath or whether you're happy to stay in the moment. Remember to stay within your comfort zone and adjust your breath, particularly the retentions, as needed to practise 'easeful effort'.

Counting the breath is also a great tool to focus your mind on the present moment; if you lose your place, you can simply start over.

PRACTICE

1. Box breathing can be practised lying down or seated, so get into a comfortable position that you can stay in for a few minutes.

2. If you feel comfortable, close your eyes or soften your gaze and let your eyelids feel heavy.

3. Take a moment to breathe normally and notice how you feel in body and mind.

4. After a few breaths, start to breathe in and out through the nose if you're not already (if you have a cold or any nasal restrictions, breathe in whatever way feels most comfortable).

5. When you're ready, start to count the breath, inhaling for two counts and exhaling for two counts.

6. As long as there are no contraindications, see if you can notice the slight pause at the end of the inhalation and the slight pause at the end of the exhalation.

7. After a few breaths, start to extend these pauses so that they last for two counts, breathing in for two, holding the breath for two, exhaling for two and holding the breath out for two.

8. Continue to breathe in this way for a few breaths, taking time to observe the effects of the practice.

9. If you feel ready, you can adjust the count to three or four, making sure to keep the breath equal. If this is too much, you can go back to breathing in and out for two counts.

10. You can practise this *pranayama* technique for as long as you're comfortable (a couple of minutes may be enough or you may continue for 10–15 minutes).

11. When you're ready to conclude the practice, return to your natural breathing and cease counting, while keeping the eyes closed.

12. Take a moment to notice how the practice has affected you in mind and body before opening your eyes.

JOURNALLING PROMPTS

* How does this advanced version of *sama vritti* compare to the equal breath practice? Do you have a preference between the two?

* How comfortable is it to hold and exhale the breath for longer counts?

* Do you visualise a box as you do this practice? If not, is visualisation something you would like to add to your practice?

Ujjayi Breath

(Victorious Breath/Ocean Breath): Advanced Version

PRECAUTIONS

* Pregnancy.

* Chronic fatigue.

* Low blood pressure.

* Hypertension.

* Heart conditions.

BENEFITS

* Slows the breath.

* Helps to calm the nervous system.

* Builds *agni* (inner fire) within the body.

* Energises mind and body.

* Stimulates the *vishuddha chakra* (throat chakra).

* Enhances mental focus and concentration.

We covered the basics of *ujjayi* breath on pages 33–5. If you have practised this a few times and feel comfortable to move onto the next stage during which the throat is restricted on the inhalation as well as the exhalation, then we will give full instructions here.

Remember, *ujjayi* breath makes a soft sound as the breath moves through the throat, hence why it is often called ocean breath. We encourage you not to force your breath; a soft sound that only you can hear is perfectly fine.

PRACTICE

Note: Ujjayi is also commonly practised when carrying out yoga *asana*, but for the purposes of this journal, we suggest you practise in stillness, at least to begin with.

1. *Ujjayi* can be practised when seated or lying down, so find a comfortable seated position that you can stay in for a few minutes.

2. Close your eyes to avoid distractions and take a moment to tune into your natural breath, noting how it feels today, in this moment.

3. Breathe in through the nose.

4. As you breathe out, open your mouth and make a soft, slow 'haa' sound. To make this sound you'll naturally restrict the throat. If you aren't sure whether you're getting this quite right, imagine you're holding a small mirror in front of your mouth and your breath out is fogging up the mirror.

5. Once you're comfortable with this, try to breathe out with the mouth closed, still restricting the throat.

6. You should notice a soft sound, a bit like the waves of the ocean.

7. Continue to breathe with the mouth closed, restricting the throat on the exhalation.

8. When you're ready, try to retain the restriction of the throat as you breathe in as well. This will create a soft sound on the inhalation as well as the exhalation.

9. Continue to breathe in this way for a couple of minutes, noticing how this change in the inhalation affects the quality of the breath. Do you find your breath slowing down or speeding up? Do you feel any physical effects in the body, particularly around the throat, upper shoulders, upper back, chest, and ribs?

10. When you're ready to complete the practice, release the restriction of the throat and breathe naturally, taking a moment to notice any changes to how you feel.

JOURNALLING PROMPTS

* How does this advanced version of *ujjayi* compare to the foundational practice? Do you have a preference between the two?

* Which physical effects, if any, did you notice while doing this practice?

* Are there times in your life when you would benefit from an energising practice like this? How might you incorporate *ujjayi* into your *pranayama* toolkit?

Nadi Shodhana (Alternate Nostril Breathing)

PRECAUTIONS

* Do not practise if you're experiencing a chronic respiratory condition.

BENEFITS

* Brings calm and balance to body and mind.

* Supports becoming more mindful of the present moment.

* Increases focus and concentration.

* Lowers heart rate.

* Balances the left and right sides of the body and brain.

* Said to purify the *nadis* (the energy channels in the body) so that energy flows more freely.

* May help to remove blockages in the nose or sinuses.

We covered the practices of *surya bhedana* and *chandra bhedana* on pages 41–6. Both are great preparation for *nadi shodhana*, also known as alternate nostril breathing. *Nadi* is a Sanskrit word meaning *flow* or *channel*, while *shodhana* means *purification* or *clearing*. This *pranayama* technique is therefore said to clear away any blockages in the energy lines, allowing *prana* (lifeforce) to flow freely through the body.

It may be interesting to journal about any imbalances within the body or mind before and after practising *nadi shodhana* to see if it has any effect.

PRACTICE

Note: For a more calming, restorative practice, start by breathing in through the left nostril.

1. This technique is usually practised while seated, so find a comfortable sitting position where you can sit upright comfortably for a few minutes.

2. Take a moment to breathe naturally and begin to pay attention to air flow in your nostrils. Is one side easier to breathe through than the other, or is it difficult to tell the difference?

3. Bring your right hand in front of your face, placing your thumb on your right nostril and your ring and little fingers on the left nostril. The middle two fingers can rest in between your eyebrows, or you can tuck them in towards the palm. The left hand can rest on your lap or on your left thigh or knee.

4. Keeping the left nostril blocked, release the right nostril and breathe in for four counts.

5. Block the right nostril with the thumb and retain the breath for four counts.

6. Release the left nostril and breathe out for four counts.

7. Pause for four counts, holding out the breath.

8. Breathe in through the left nostril for a count of four.

9. Block both nostrils and hold for four counts.

10. Breathe out through the right nostril for four counts.

11. Repeat steps 4–10 as many times as you're comfortable for 5–10 minutes.

12. When you're ready to conclude the practice, exhale through the right nostril, release the hand, and take a few breaths through both nostrils. Think back to the observations you made in step 2 and notice whether there has been any change.

You can explore variations on this advanced practice for yourself once you're familiar with the basics. Here are some ideas to get you started:

* Breathe in through one nostril and out through the other.

* Breathe in and out through one nostril, then swap sides.

* Breathe in and out through the same nostril more than once before swapping sides.

* Experiment with retaining the breath before swapping sides.

JOURNALLING PROMPTS

* Did you explore *nadi shodhana* with the suggestions above? Is there a way of doing this practice that resonates most with you?

* What changes do you notice in yourself after completing this practice?

* Are there times when you feel stuck in a rut or that you have a creative block? How might you use *nadi shodhana* as part of your *pranayama* toolkit?

Sun Breath: Linking Breath to Movement

PRECAUTIONS

∗ None.

BENEFITS

∗ Activates the parasympathetic nervous system, so very effective for anxiety and stress.

∗ Regulates the breath.

Many of the *pranayama* practices in this journal are practised in stillness, but sitting still in one position can prove to be challenging if you aren't used to it. Therefore, we have included the following practice, the sun breath, which links very simple movements with the breath.

If you find that you have a lot of thoughts running through your head and find it difficult to focus, then this practice is for you! Adding the element of movement gives your mind something additional to focus on, hopefully making it a little easier to concentrate on your practice. This type of breathing also activates the parasympathetic nervous system (the rest and digest response – see page 37 for more details). For these reasons, the sun breath can work particularly well for people who are experiencing anxiety or stress.

We've given two options for how to move the hands when practising the sun breath. You may prefer one over the other, which is, of course, absolutely fine. Once you have practised this a few times, you may wish to experiment with the movements of the hands and the arms in conjunction with the breath. Be sure to make a note of what you try and what does and doesn't feel good for you in your journal.

PRACTICE #1

1. This technique is usually practised while seated, so find a comfortable sitting position where you can sit upright comfortably for a few minutes.

2. Breathe naturally and begin to note the qualities of your breath (breath awareness) and your state of mind.

3. If it feels comfortable, begin to breathe in and out through the nose if you aren't already.

4. Place your hands on your knees, palms facing down and close your eyes or lower your gaze.

5. When you're ready, breathe in and slowly lift both hands away from the knees by a few inches. You don't need to lift them very far.

6. As you breathe out, slowly lower your hands so they're almost touching your knees.

7. Continue to breathe in and out this way for a few minutes, lifting your hands as you inhale and lowering them as you exhale. This can be a very small, subtle movement, but try not to allow your hands to touch your knees.

8. As you're practising, begin to pay attention to the palms of your hands and notice any sensations that may arise.

9. When you're ready to conclude the practice, place your palms onto your knees and take a few natural breaths before opening your eyes.

PRACTICE #2

1. This technique is usually practised while seated, so find a comfortable

sitting position where you can sit upright comfortably for a few minutes.

2. Breathe naturally and begin to note the qualities of your breath (breath awareness) and your state of mind.

3. If it feels comfortable, begin to breathe in and out through the nose if you aren't already.

4. Bring your hands to *anjali mudra* (prayer position) in front of your chest (your *anahata chakra* or heart centre) and close your eyes or lower your gaze.

5. When you're ready, breathe in and slowly separate your hands. You can take your arms as wide as feels comfortable.

6. As you breathe out, bring your hands closer together so that they're almost touching in *anjali mudra* in front of the chest, but not quite.

7. Continue to breathe in and out this way for a few minutes, separating your hands as you inhale and bringing them towards your heart centre as you exhale. This can be a very small, subtle movement, but try not to allow your hands to touch each other.

8. As you're practising, begin to pay attention to the palms of your hands and notice any sensations that may arise.

9. When you're ready to conclude the practice, bring your hands back to *anjali mudra* and take a few natural breaths before opening your eyes.

JOURNALLING PROMPTS

*   If you're feeling anxious or stressed, it may be useful to write some notes in your journal about how you're feeling before and after this

practice so that you can see if there are any subtle differences in the way you feel after practising.

* How do you feel in your mind and body after this practice?

* Does your natural breath feel any different?

* Did you notice any physical sensations, particularly in the hands or heart, during this practice?

* Are there any other small, simple movements that you could experiment with while practising *pranayama*? If you adapt your practice, be sure to make a note so that you can remember which movements felt good.

Dirga Pranayama (Three-Part Yogic Breath/Jug Breath)

PRECAUTIONS

* The inhalation and any pause (or retention) should not be longer than the exhalation as this affects blood pressure.

BENEFITS

* Can calm the nervous system and reduce anxiety.

* Increases lung capacity.

* Focuses the mind.

* Lowers heart rate and blood pressure.

* Reduces insomnia.

In this *pranayama* practice, we split both the inhalation and exhalation into three parts. This can take a little bit of getting used to, especially if you're new to *pranayama*. However, many people find this practice very grounding and calming, so try to persevere if you find it tricky, as the rewards are worth it.

Dirga is the Sanskrit word for *complete and long,* reflecting the fullness of the breath in this practice. *Dirga pranayama* encourages using our full lung capacity, envisaging the lungs filling completely from top to bottom. Some people like to imagine the lungs as being like a big jug that we gradually fill with breath in three stages, then empty out, again, in three stages.

To make this practice more accessible, we begin by splitting the breath into two parts, then progressing to three parts, if you feel comfortable. We start by splitting the exhalation into two parts – this anchors the breath

– then we split the inhalation into parts, then finally we put everything together. You may wish to stick to a two-part breath, or just stick to splitting the inhalation or exhalation only. This is a great way to get started and we encourage you to experiment with this *pranayama* exercise to find a practice that feels right for you. Your journal will be useful here; as you practise over the course of several weeks you might start to notice that you're utilising more of your lung capacity and taking a deeper breath, or that you find it easier to breathe in this way.

PRACTICE

1. This practice can be done seated or lying down, so make yourself comfortable and find a position to sit or lie in where you can stay for a few minutes.

2. Close your eyes or soften your gaze.

3. Take a few moments to notice your natural breath and ask yourself how you're feeling today, in this precise moment.

4. If possible, begin to breathe in and out through the nose if you aren't already.

5. When you're ready to begin, exhale in two parts: breathe out half-way, take a slight pause and then breathe out the remaining breath.

6. Inhale naturally.

7. Repeat steps 5 and 6 for a few rounds of breath, exhaling in two stages, and inhaling naturally.

8. Next, breathe out, keeping the exhalation longer than the inhalation.

9. Inhale in two parts; breathing in halfway, taking a slight pause, then breathing in further to fill the lungs.

10. Continue to breathe in this way, repeating steps 8 and 9 as many times as you like.

11. Next, try exhaling in three parts. Release one third of the breath, pause, release another third and pause, then release the remaining third. Inhale naturally.

12. Continue to breathe in this way for a few rounds of breath, repeating steps 11 and 12 as many times as you like.

13. Then, breathe naturally.

14. Next, try inhaling in three parts. Visualise your lungs as a big pot that you're filling with air. Breathe in a third of the way, pause, then breathe in another third of the way, pause, then breathe in the remaining third of the way to fill the lungs.

15. Continue to breathe in this way for a few rounds of breath, repeating steps 14 and 15 as many times as you like.

16. When you're ready to put everything together, exhale in three parts and inhale in three parts. If this is tricky, start by splitting the inhalation and exhalation into two parts first and progress to a three-part breath, if and when you feel comfortable to do so.

17. When you're ready to conclude your practice, come back to your natural breath. Take some time to note how your breath feels in the moment and how you feel in the body and mind.

18. Open your eyes.

JOURNALLING PROMPTS

* How did you find the three-part yogic breath practice? How did it make you feel?

*   Did you prefer splitting up the breath into parts on the inhalation or the exhalation?

*   Were you more comfortable splitting the breath into two or three parts?

*   Did you like visualising the lungs as a pot filling with air? Is there something else that you visualised that you found useful to guide you through the practice?

*   If you're practising this over several weeks, take a moment to look back through your notes to see if anything has changed. Do you feel calmer and more grounded? More energised? Or perhaps more focused and present?

Kapalabhati (Skull-Shining Breath)

PRECAUTIONS

* Don't practise *kapalabhati* on a full stomach!

* Pregnancy.

This practice isn't suitable for people who are managing a number of chronic conditions or experiencing any of the following:

* dizziness

* high blood pressure

* epilepsy

* migraine

* stomach or intestinal ulcers

* hernias

* brain tumours

* stroke

* heart disease

* GERD

* gastritis

* glaucoma

* diarrhoea

* systemic inflammation

* hyperventilation.

BENEFITS

* Improves circulation.

* Improves mental focus and concentration.

* Increases lung strength and function.

* Clears the nasal passages.

* Tones the abdominal muscles.

Strictly speaking, *kapalabhati* is a *kriya* (an internal cleansing practice) but we have included it here because, essentially, it is a breathing practice too.

Kapalabhati has quite different benefits to many of the *pranayama* techniques covered in this book, which are included to promote relaxation. Unlike most of the other practices in the journal, it can be done rapidly and can have a very energising effect on the body. Also, the inhalation is passive, meaning it occurs naturally after a forceful exhalation. Therefore, it is best practised earlier in the day, and it should be practised on an empty stomach as it works the abdominal muscles.

The word *kapala* means skull and *bhati* means illuminating, so *kapalabhati* is often called the skull-shining breath. It is said that practising *kapalabhati* regularly will make the forehead luminous. The *ajna chakra* is located in the centre of the forehead and is said to be the centre of intuition and inner knowledge. Therefore, this energy centre is said to be activated by regular practice of *kapalabhati*.

PRACTICE

Note: You may wish to blow your nose before you begin this practice.

1. *Kapalabhati* is best practised while seated with an upright spine, so come to sit in *sukhasana* (cross-legged) or *vajrasana* (kneeling).

2. Close your eyes or soften your gaze and start to breathe in and out through your nose if you aren't already.

3. Breathe in through the nose.

4. Exhale forcefully through your nose while at the same time contracting the abdominal muscles. You may make a sniffing sound on the exhalation. You'll find that you only need to focus on the exhalation as the inhalation will happen naturally.

5. Continue to breathe in this way, keeping the spine upright and trying to minimise movement in the shoulders and chest.

6. Complete 27 rounds of *kapalabhati*.

7. When you're ready to complete the practice, take a deep breath in followed by a deep breath out.

8. Take a moment to notice the effects of the practice.

9. Repeat the practice up to three times if you wish, remembering to take a break in between rounds.

JOURNALLING PROMPTS

* How do you feel after this practice? How did it differ from some of the other techniques you have tried?

* Did you notice any physical sensations during or after this practice?

* How did the practice affect your energy levels?

MUDRAS

Mudras are positions or gestures, usually made with the hands and fingers, which can be practised alongside *pranayama* exercises. In the yoga tradition, *mudras* are said to further stimulate and direct *prana* and offer a point of focus for the mind, making them an ideal accompaniment to *pranayama*. Here we have included a few common *mudras* to try and incorporate into your practice.

Chin Mudra (Gesture of Consciousness)

PRECAUTIONS

* None.

BENEFITS

* Aids concentration.

* Can help you feel calm and grounded.

* Helps with depression.

* Opens the lower part of the lungs.

Chin mudra is one of the most commonly used *mudras*. Its name means *gesture of consciousness* and it's often used to cultivate concentration. In this *mudra,* we join the index finger (representing individual consciousness) and the thumb (representing universal consciousness). This *mudra* is said to unite these two aspects of our consciousness.

Chin mudra is very similar to *jnana mudra* (gesture of wisdom) – the hand positions are the same – but in *chin mudra* the palms face downwards (for grounding and calming) and in *jnana mudra* the palms face upwards (for openness and enquiry). You may wish to explore both options during your practice and journal about the effects these *mudras* have on you.

PRACTICE

1. *Chin mudra* can be practised in any position, but we recommend beginning with a seated practice. So come to a comfortable sitting position that you can stay in for a few minutes.

2. Close your eyes or soften your gaze and breathe in and out through the nose if you aren't already.

3. To take *chin mudra*, lightly join the tip of your thumb and the tip of your first finger on each hand and place your hands on your knees with the palms facing down. The remaining fingers should be extended but relaxed.

4. Continue to breathe with your hands in this *mudra*, taking time to feel into the subtle feelings and sensations of your breath, body, and mind.

5. You can continue to practise in this way for as long as you like.

6. When you're ready to complete the practice, relax your hands to release the *mudra* and take a few comfortable breaths before opening your eyes.

Brahma Mudra (Gesture of Supreme Spirit)

PRECAUTIONS

∗   Arthritis or pain in the hands.

BENEFITS

∗   Revitalises the whole system.

∗   Encourages deeper breathing.

∗   Promotes a sense of calm.

∗   Stimulates the digestive system.

Brahma, which means supreme in Sanskrit, is the creator of the universe, hence this mudra is often known as the gesture of supreme spirit. When making this gesture of the hands alongside pranayama, the mudra is said to encourage full, deep breaths and can therefore leave us feeling calm and relaxed. Because the hands are placed at the manipura chakra (the chakra that focuses on our inner fire), this gesture is said to activate our agni, which is why it is said to stimulate digestion.

PRACTICE

1. Brahma mudra is usually held when seated, so come to a comfortable sitting position that you can stay in for a few minutes and where the spine is upright.

2. Close your eyes or soften your gaze and begin to breathe in and out through the nose, if you aren't already.

3. On each hand, tuck your thumb and then curl your fingers around it. Face your palms up and bring your knuckles together to touch

in front of *manipura chakra*, the point where your lower ribs meet. Keep your shoulders and arms relaxed.

4. Continue to breathe while maintaining the *mudra*, noticing how you feel both physically and emotionally. You can continue to breathe in this way for as long as is comfortable.

5. When you're ready to conclude the practice, allow your hands to soften and release the *mudra*.

6. Take a few more breaths and eventually open your eyes.

Kali Mudra (Gesture of the Goddess Kali)

PRECAUTIONS

* None.

BENEFITS

* Said to improve the effects of depression, anxiety, and insomnia, bringing a greater sense of energy, ease, and relaxation.

* Clears blockages in the *sushumna nadi* (central channel).

* Reduces physical, mental, and emotional tension.

Kali mudra is a commonly used *mudra* and is said to represent the Hindu goddess Kali, who represents embodied inner strength and empowerment. It has many benefits but, most importantly, it is said to promote a feeling of calmness in the body while releasing blocked *prana* in the energy channels. The position of the hands, with the index fingers pointing away from the body, can be said to represent a pouring away or letting go, so it can be helpful to visualise releasing anything that doesn't serve you when undertaking this practice.

PRACTICE

1. *Kali mudra* can be done when seated or reclined, so come to a comfortable position that you can stay in for a few minutes and where the spine is lengthened.

2. Close your eyes or soften the gaze and begin to breathe in and out through the nose if you aren't already.

3. Interlace all ten fingers and release both index fingers. Your thumbs

should remain crossed as the index fingers, making a pointing gesture.

4. Bring the *mudra* to your lap with your index fingers pointing away from you, making sure your arms and shoulders are relaxed.

5. Continue to breathe while maintaining the *mudra,* noticing how you feel both physically and emotionally. You can continue to breathe in this way for up to 10 minutes.

6. When you're ready to conclude the practice, allow your hands to soften and release the *mudra.*

7. Take a few more breaths and eventually open your eyes.

JOURNALLING PROMPTS

* Did you notice any energetic effects from breathing during or after the practice?

* Did you feel any physical effects?

* Which *mudra* did you prefer to use?

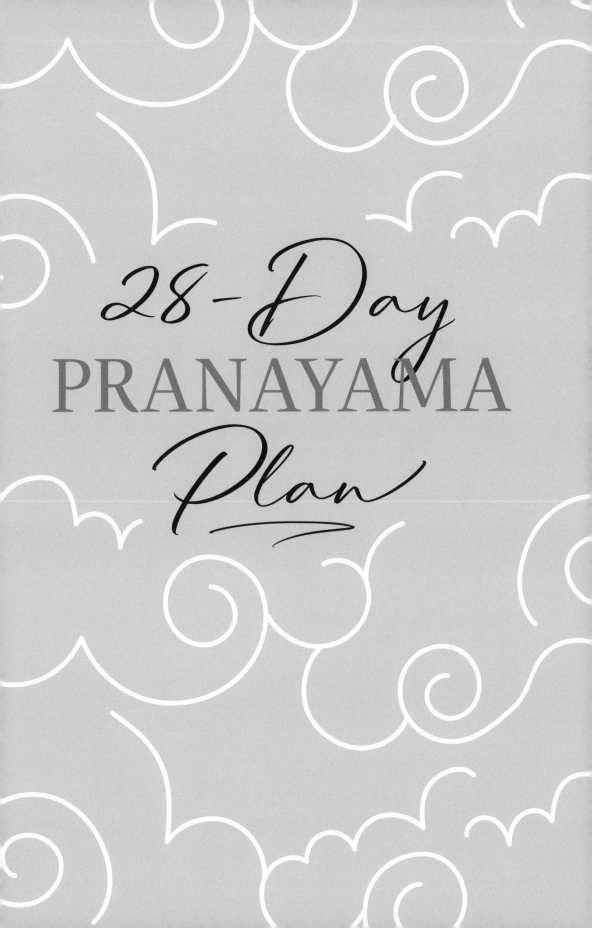

28-Day
PRANAYAMA
Plan

In this section, we have included a daily practice plan. Remember, these are merely invitations and suggestions to practise, and you should feel free to adjust your practice as needed. We have also suggested timings for each day's practice, but you can practise for longer than this if you'd like.

For the first week, we have repeated the practice instructions to help you become familiar with the techniques.

Remember, you can access audio recordings of all of the *pranayama* techniques at https://library.jkp.com/redeem using the code WLDEQJK. You may find it easier to practise the techniques alongside the recordings at first, then eventually start to practise on your own.

Week 1

FOUNDATIONAL TECHNIQUES

Day 1

SUGGESTED PRACTICE

* Breath awareness

SUGGESTED PRACTICE TIME

🕑 5 minutes

PRACTICE

1. Breath awareness can be practised lying down or seated, so get into a comfortable position that you can stay in for a few minutes.

2. If you feel comfortable, close your eyes or soften your gaze and let your eyelids feel heavy.

3. Breathe naturally, trying not to manipulate the breath or control it in any way.

4. Once you're settled into a natural breath, take a moment to notice whether you're breathing in and out through the mouth or nose. Perhaps you're breathing in through the nose and out through the mouth, or vice versa. Or maybe you're breathing in and out through the nose, or just through the mouth. Don't try to change anything; just notice what comes naturally.

5. Now, begin to pay attention to where the breath enters and leaves the body, either through the nose or mouth. Does the temperature of the air coming in feel cooler or warmer going out?

6. Take some time to be curious about the quality of your breathing. Is it fast or slow, is the inhalation longer or shorter than the exhalation? Does the breath feel smooth and comfortable, or does it feel restricted in any way? Is it more comfortable to breathe in or breathe out, or perhaps you find both the same?

7. Then, when you're ready, start to bring your awareness to where you feel the physical effects of the breath in the body. You might feel movements or sensations in the throat, nasal passage, shoulders, chest, ribs, or belly. You might even feel something in the hands or feet. Take your time here to notice your unique experience of the breath.

8. Next, begin to notice how your breathing makes you feel energetically or emotionally. Do you feel calm and comfortable, or do you feel anxious or stressed? Or perhaps you're somewhere in between, or you aren't quite sure. There is no right answer; just go with what comes up.

9. If at any point, your thoughts start to intrude on your breath awareness practice, go back to one of the earlier steps. It is perfectly normal for our minds to start thinking about something else.

10. To conclude the practice, bring your focus back to your natural breath and make a mental note as to whether you notice anything different.

JOURNALLING PROMPTS

*   What did you notice about your breath at the start of your practice

today? Were you naturally breathing through the nose or the mouth? Was the breath fast or slow? Calm or laboured?

* How easy did you find it to maintain a focus on your breathing? Did you get easily distracted, or was it easy to maintain your focus once you got started?

* How did you feel at the end of the practice? Were there any differences in your breathing compared to the start of the practice?

Day 2

SUGGESTED PRACTICE

* *Sama vritti* (equal breathing): beginner's version

SUGGESTED PRACTICE TIME

🕐 5 minutes

PRACTICE

1. *Sama vritti* can be practised lying down or seated, so get into a comfortable position that you can stay in for a few minutes.

2. If you feel comfortable, close your eyes or soften your gaze and let your eyelids feel heavy.

3. Take a moment to breathe naturally and notice how you feel in body and mind.

4. After a few breaths, start to breathe in and out through the nose if you aren't already. If you have a cold or any nasal restrictions, breathe in whatever way feels most comfortable.

5. When you're ready, start to count the breath, inhaling for two counts and exhaling for two counts.

6. As long as there are no contraindications, see if you can notice the slight pause at the end of the inhalation and the slight pause at the end of the exhalation.

7. Continue to breathe in this way for a few breaths, taking time to observe the effects of the practice.

8. If you feel ready, you can adjust the count to three or four, making sure to keep the breath equal. If it's too much, you can go back to breathing in and out for two counts.

9. When you're ready to conclude the practice, stop counting and return to your natural breath, taking some time to notice the after-effects of the *pranayama*.

JOURNALLING PROMPTS

* How did you find today's practice? Did you find it easy to breathe in and out for equal counts?

* If this was challenging, what part of the breath did you find more tricky, the inhalation or the exhalation?

* Did you try adjusting the counts and, if so, how did that go?

* How did you feel at the end of the practice?

* Is there anything you would like to do differently next time?

Day 3

SUGGESTED PRACTICES

* Breath awareness

* *Simhasana pranayama* (lion's breath)

SUGGESTED PRACTICE TIME

🕐 5 minutes

Note: You may find it tricky to practise lion's breath for up to 5 minutes, so here we suggest combining with breath awareness or another simple practice.

PRACTICE: BREATH AWARENESS

1. Breath awareness can be practised lying down or seated, so get into a comfortable position that you can stay in for a few minutes.

2. If you feel comfortable, close your eyes or soften your gaze and let your eyelids feel heavy.

3. Breathe naturally, trying not to manipulate the breath or control it in any way.

4. Once you're settled into a natural breath, take a moment to notice whether you're breathing in and out through the mouth or nose. Perhaps you're breathing in through the nose and out through the mouth, or vice versa. Or maybe you're breathing in and out through the nose, or just through the mouth. Don't try to change anything; just notice what comes naturally.

5. Now begin to pay attention to where the breath enters and leaves

the body, either through the nose or mouth. Does the temperature of the air coming in feel cooler or warmer going out?

6. Take some time to be curious about the quality of your breathing. Is it fast or slow? Is the inhalation longer or shorter than the exhalation? Does the breath feel smooth and comfortable, or does it feel restricted in any way? Is it more comfortable to breathe in or breathe out, or perhaps you find both the same?

7. Then, when you're ready, start to bring your awareness to where you feel the physical effects of the breath in the body. You might feel movements or sensations in the throat, nasal passage, shoulders, chest, ribs, or belly. You might even feel something in the hands or feet. Take your time here to notice your unique experience of the breath.

8. Next, begin to notice how your breathing makes you feel energetically or emotionally. Do you feel calm and comfortable, or do you feel anxious or stressed? Or perhaps you're somewhere in between, or you aren't quite sure. There is no right answer; just go with what comes up.

9. If at any point, your thoughts start to intrude on your breath awareness practice, go back to one of the earlier steps. It is perfectly normal for our minds to start thinking about something else.

10. To conclude the practice, bring your focus back to your natural breath and make a mental note as to whether you notice anything different.

PRACTICE: SIMHASANA PRANAYAMA (LION'S BREATH)

1. Lion's breath is best practised while seated, so either come to a comfortable seated position or sit kneeling with the knees wide and the big toes touching.

2. Take a moment to become aware of your breath, taking a few comfortable, nourishing breaths to settle your body and mind.

3. Open your eyes and breathe in through the nose.

4. If you're kneeling, place your hands in front of you with the palms facing down, fingertips pointed towards you (the wrists are facing forwards).

5. Open your eyes wide with your gaze focused on the point between your eyebrows (this is also known as *ajna chakra*, the third eye point). If you're kneeling, lean forwards on the exhale, keeping the back straight. However, if you're sitting, exhale through the mouth, sticking your tongue out as far as you can. As you exhale, make a 'hahhh' sound, a bit like a lion's roar.

6. Repeat twice more.

7. Come back to your natural breath, taking a moment to notice the effects of the practice. You can repeat this practice if you wish.

JOURNALLING PROMPTS

* What did you notice about your breath at the start of your practice today? Were you naturally breathing through the nose or the mouth? Was the breath fast or slow? Calm or laboured?

* What was your experience physically and emotionally when practising these techniques?

* How did it feel to use the sound of your breath in your practice?

* How did you feel at the end of the practice? Were there any differences in your breathing compared to the start of the practice?

Day 4

SUGGESTED PRACTICE

*   *Ujjayi* breath (victorious breath/ocean breath): beginner's version

SUGGESTED PRACTICE TIME

🕐 5 minutes

PRACTICE

1. *Ujjayi* can be done when seated or lying down, so find a comfortable seated position that you can stay in for a few minutes.

2. Close your eyes to avoid distractions and take a moment to tune into your natural breath, noting how it feels today, in this moment.

3. Breathe in through your nose.

4. As you breathe out, open your mouth and make a soft, slow 'haa' sound. To make this sound, you'll naturally restrict the throat. If you aren't sure you're getting this quite right, imagine you're holding a small mirror in front of your mouth and your breath out is fogging up the mirror.

5. Once you're comfortable with this, try to breathe out with the mouth closed, still restricting the throat.

6. You should notice a soft sound, a bit like the waves of the ocean.

7. Continue to breathe with the mouth closed, restricting the throat on the exhalation.

8. When you're ready to complete the practice of *ujjayi*, release the

restriction of the throat and breathe naturally, taking a moment to notice any changes to how you feel.

JOURNALLING PROMPTS

✳ Is this *pranayama* technique new to you or something you have tried in the past? If you've done this before, did the experience feel any different? How so?

✳ Did you notice any changes in the length of your exhalation once you started to use the throat to create the *ujjayi* breath? Did you notice anything else?

✳ Did you find it comfortable to breathe in this way? If not, what were the challenges?

✳ How focused did you feel in your practice today? If it's helpful, you can give yourself a score out of 10, 10 being very focused and 1 finding it very difficult to maintain your focus on your breathwork practice. Try not to get competitive or feel frustrated if you have some days when the focus was not as forthcoming. Just observe these frustrations and know that you can try again later.

Day 5

SUGGESTED PRACTICE

✳ Extended exhalation

SUGGESTED PRACTICE TIME

🕐 5 minutes

PRACTICE

1. This practice can be done seated or lying down, so make yourself comfortable and find a position to sit or lie in where you can stay for a few minutes.

2. Close your eyes or soften your gaze.

3. Take a few moments to notice your natural breath and ask yourself how you're feeling today, in this precise moment.

4. If possible, begin to breathe in and out through the nose if you're not already.

5. When you're ready, start to count the breath, breathing in for a count of two and out for a count of two.

6. Take a few even, equal breaths and when you're ready you can start to extend the exhalation, breathing in for two and breathing out for three or even four counts.

7. Continue to breathe in this way for at least 2 minutes if you can. You can even make the exhalation longer if you wish. The breath should not feel forced or uncomfortable in any way.

8. When you're ready to conclude the practice, come back to your natural breath and cease counting.

9. Take a moment to note how you feel in both body and mind.

10. This practice can be repeated at any point during your day.

JOURNALLING PROMPTS

* How did you feel at the start of this practice? How did you feel by the end of this practice?

* Did anything unexpected come up for you during this practice? If so, observe how this makes you feel without judgement.

* Are there times in your life when this practice might be particularly useful? If so, remember that this practice is part of your toolkit and that you can return to it at any time.

Day 6

SUGGESTED PRACTICE

✳ *Surya bhedana* (alternate nostril breathing/sun-piercing breath)

SUGGESTED PRACTICE TIME

🕐 5 minutes

Note: Surya bhedana is an energising practice, so best practised in the morning or when you need to increase energy levels.

PRACTICE

1. This technique is usually practised while seated, so find a comfortable sitting position where you can sit upright comfortably for a few minutes.

2. Take a moment to breathe naturally and begin to pay attention to your nostrils. Is one side of your nose easier to breathe through than the other, or is it difficult to tell the difference?

3. Bring your right hand in front of your face, placing your thumb on your right nostril and your ring and little fingers on the left nostril. The middle two fingers can rest in between your eyebrows, or you can tuck them in towards the palm. Your left hand can rest on your lap or on your left thigh or knee.

4. Keeping the left nostril blocked, release the right nostril and breathe in.

5. Block the right nostril with the thumb, release the left nostril and breathe out.

6. Repeat, breathing in through the right nostril and out through the left nostril.

7. When you're ready to conclude the practice, release your hand and take a few breaths through both nostrils. Think back to the observations you made in step 2 and notice whether there has been any change.

JOURNALLING PROMPTS

* What time of day is it? How do you usually feel at this time, without having done this practice?

* Now that you have done this practice, what changes do you notice in yourself? It's ok if you don't feel more energised after the first attempt; you can simply try again later.

* How comfortable was your breath during this practice?

Day 7

* *Chandra bhedana* (alternate nostril breathing/moon-piercing breath)

SUGGESTED PRACTICE TIME

🕐 5 minutes

Note: Chandra bhedana is a calming practice, so best practised in the evening or before bed.

PRACTICE

1. This technique is usually practised while seated, so find a comfortable sitting position where you can sit upright comfortably for a few minutes.

2. Take a moment to breathe naturally and begin to pay attention to your nostrils. Is one side easier to breathe through than the other, or is it difficult to tell the difference?

3. Bring your right hand in front of your face, placing your thumb on your right nostril and your ring and little fingers on the left nostril. The middle two fingers can rest in between your eyebrows, or you can tuck them in towards the palm. Your left hand can rest on your lap or on your left thigh or knee.

4. Keeping the right nostril blocked, release the left nostril and breathe in.

5. Block the left nostril with the thumb, release the right nostril and breathe out.

6. Repeat, breathing in through the left nostril and out through the right nostril.

7. When you're ready to conclude the practice, release your hand and take a few breaths through both nostrils. Think back to the observations you made in step 2 and notice whether there has been any change.

JOURNALLING PROMPTS

∗ What time of day is it? How do you usually feel at this time, without having done this practice?

∗ Now that you have done this practice, what changes do you notice in yourself? It's ok if you don't feel calmer after the first attempt; you can simply try again later.

∗ How comfortable was your breath during this practice? How does it compare to sun-piercing breath?

Week 2

INTERMEDIATE TECHNIQUES

Day 8

SUGGESTED PRACTICES

*   Breath awareness

*   *Sama vritti* (equal breathing): beginner's version

*   *Sitali pranayama* (cooling breath)

SUGGESTED PRACTICE TIME

🕐 5–10 minutes

Note: Sitali pranayama is a cooling practice so we suggest practising for up to 2 minutes and if the weather is very cold you may prefer to choose a more warming practice such as *ujjayi*.

Day 9

SUGGESTED PRACTICES

* Breath awareness

* *Bhramari pranayama* (bee breath)

SUGGESTED PRACTICE TIME

🕐 5–10 minutes

Day 10

SUGGESTED PRACTICES

* Breath awareness

* *Sama vritti* (equal breathing): beginner's version

SUGGESTED PRACTICE TIME

🕐 5–10 minutes

Day 11

SUGGESTED PRACTICES

* Breath awareness

* *Ujjayi* breath (victorious breath/ocean breath): beginner's version

SUGGESTED PRACTICE TIME

🕐 5–10 minutes

Day 12

SUGGESTED PRACTICES

* Breath awareness

* *Simhasana pranayama* (lion's breath)

SUGGESTED PRACTICE TIME

🕐 5–10 minutes

Day 13

SUGGESTED PRACTICES

✳ Extended exhalation

✳ *Sitali pranayama* (cooling breath)

SUGGESTED PRACTICE TIME

🕐 5–10 minutes

Note: Sitali pranayama is a cooling practice so we suggest practising for up to 2 minutes and if the weather is very cold you may prefer to choose a more warming practice such as lion's breath.

Day 14

SUGGESTED PRACTICES

✳ Extended exhalation

✳ *Bhramari pranayama* (bee breath)

SUGGESTED PRACTICE TIME

🕐 5–10 minutes

Week 3

ADVANCED TECHNIQUES

Day 15

SUGGESTED PRACTICE

✳ *Sama vritti* (box breathing): advanced version

SUGGESTED PRACTICE TIME

🕐 5 minutes

Day 16

SUGGESTED PRACTICE

* *Ujjayi* breath (victorious breath/ocean breath): advanced version

SUGGESTED PRACTICE TIME

🕐 5 minutes

Day 17

SUGGESTED PRACTICE

* *Nadi shodhana* (alternate nostril breathing): advanced version

SUGGESTED PRACTICE TIME

🕐 5 minutes

Day 18

SUGGESTED PRACTICE

* Sun breath (linking breath to movement)

SUGGESTED PRACTICE TIME

🕐 5 minutes

Day 19

SUGGESTED PRACTICE

* *Dirga pranayama* (three-part yogic breath/jug breath)

SUGGESTED PRACTICE TIME

🕐 5 minutes

WEEK 3

Day 20

SUGGESTED PRACTICES

* Breath awareness

* *Kapalabhati* (skull-shining breath)

SUGGESTED PRACTICE TIME

🕐 5 minutes – practise in the morning

Day 21

SUGGESTED PRACTICES

* Breath awareness

* *Surya bhedana* (sun-piercing breath)

SUGGESTED PRACTICE TIME

🕐 5–10 minutes – practise in the morning

Week 4

PUTTING IT ALL TOGETHER: PRANAYAMA SEQUENCES

Day 22

SUGGESTED PRACTICES

* Breath awareness

* *Chandra bhedana* (moon-piercing breath)

SUGGESTED PRACTICE TIME

🕐 10 minutes – practise in the evening

Day 23

SUGGESTED PRACTICES

* *Sama vritti* (box breathing): advanced version

* *Ujjayi* breath (victorious breath/ocean breath): advanced version

SUGGESTED PRACTICE TIME

10 minutes

Day 24

SUGGESTED PRACTICES

* *Sama vritti* (box breathing): advanced version

* Sun breath

* *Dirga pranayama* (three-part breath/jug breath)

SUGGESTED PRACTICE TIME

🕐 10–15 minutes

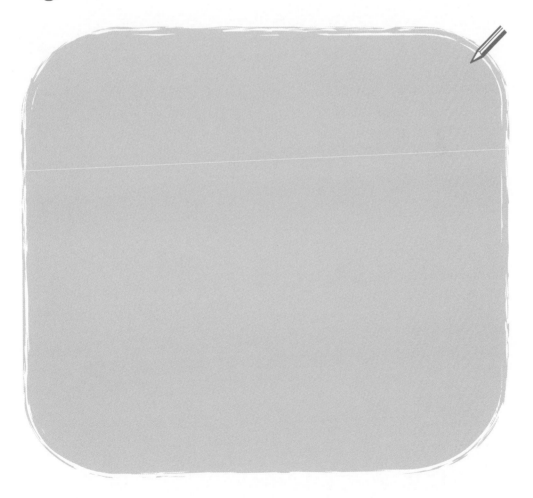

Day 25

SUGGESTED PRACTICE

✳ *Kapalabhati* (skull-shining breath)

✳ *Sama vritti* (box breathing): advanced version

✳ *Ujjayi* breath (victorious breath/ocean breath): advanced version

SUGGESTED PRACTICE TIME

🕐 10–15 minutes

Day 26

SUGGESTED PRACTICE

* *Sama vritti* (equal breathing): beginner's version

* *Bhramari pranayama* (bee breath)

* *Nadi shodhana* (alternate nostril breathing): advanced version

* Sun breath

SUGGESTED PRACTICE TIME

🕐 15 minutes

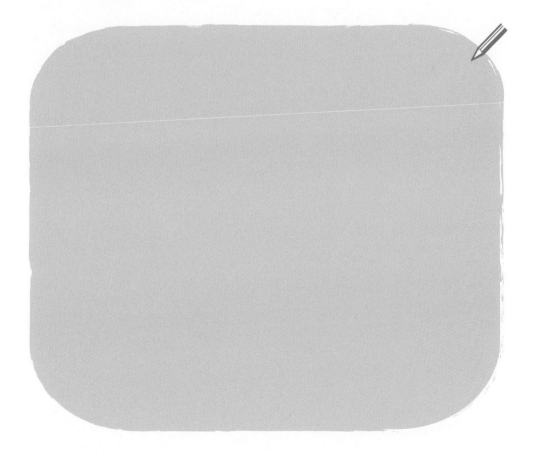

Day 27

SUGGESTED PRACTICE

* Freestyle – choose your favourite practices

SUGGESTED PRACTICE TIME

🕐 15 minutes

Day 28

SUGGESTED PRACTICE

*   Freestyle – choose your favourite practices

SUGGESTED PRACTICE TIME

🕐   15 minutes

NOTES AND OBSERVATIONS FROM WEEK 4

MAINTAINING A PRACTICE

Congratulations on completing this four-week guided journal! If you haven't already done so, take a look at your journal notes from Week 1. How do they compare to your notes from Week 4? Did anything unexpected come up? What would you like to leave behind, and what would you like to take forward into your regular practice? Ideally, these practices will now form a part of your daily routine. If not, why not try repeating one or two weeks, or adjusting the time of day you have set out to practise? Remember that you can return to this book at any time to remind yourself of the range of practices available to you.

In the next section you'll find some helpful resources to help you deepen and develop your practice.

Further Resources

❧ BOOKS ❧

Pranayama and Breathwork

Restoring Prana: A Therapeutic Guide to Pranayama and Healing Through the Breath for Yoga Therapists, Yoga Teachers, and Healthcare Practitioners, Robin L. Rothenberg (Singing Dragon)

Svadhyaya Breath Journal: A Companion Workbook to Restoring Prana, Robin L. Rothenberg (Singing Dragon)

Cultivating a Regular Practice

Developing a Yoga Home Practice: An Exploration for Yoga Teachers and Trainees, Alison Leighton with Joe Taft (Singing Dragon)

Atomic Habits: An Easy and Proven Way to Build Good Habits and Break Bad Ones, James Clear (Penguin)

Ayurveda

Ayurveda: Ancient Wisdom for Modern Wellbeing, Geeta Vara (Orion Spring)

Prajna: Ayurvedic Rituals for Happiness, Mira Manek (Headline Home)

Practical Ayurveda: Find Out Who You Are and What You Need to Bring Balance to Your Life, Sivananda Yoga Vedanta Centre (DK)

Mudras

The Healing Power of Mudras: The Yoga of the Hands, Rajendar Menen (Singing Dragon)

Mudras of Yoga: 72 Hand Gestures for Healing and Spiritual Growth, Cain Carroll with Revital Carroll (Singing Dragon, card set)

Glossary

agni Inner fire.

asana Yoga pose.

Ayurveda Translates as 'knowledge of life'. An ancient medical system with roots in India, often referred to as yoga's 'sister science'.

Bhramari pranayama Bee breath.

chakra Wheel, referring to the seven energy centres in the body (*muladhara* – root *chakra*; *svadhishthana* – sacral *chakra*; *manipura* – solar plexus *chakra*; *anahata* – heart *chakra*; *vishuddha* – throat *chakra*; *ajna* – third eye *chakra*; *sahasrara* – crown *chakra*). Each *chakra* is said to have its own related colour, shape, element, and chant.

chandra bhedana Moon-piercing breath. A breathing practice that focuses on the left nostril. Practised together with *surya bhedana,* it forms alternate nostril breathing.

dirga pranayama Three-part yogic breath or jug breath.

dosha Constitution of the body and mind. There are three *doshas*: *kapha* (associated with stability and earth and water elements); *pitta* (associated with intensity and the fire element); and *vata* (associated with creativity and air elements).

guna Quality or attribute. There are said to be three *gunas* that make up all beings: *rajas* – action; *sattva* – balance; and *tamas* – inertia.

kapalabhati Skull-shining breath.

kosha Sheath or layer. In the yoga tradition, every person is made up of five *koshas*: *annamaya* – physical layer; *pranamaya* – energetic layer; *manomaya* – mental layer; *vijnanamaya* – wisdom layer; and *anandamaya* – bliss layer.

kriya An internal cleansing practice usually carried out to achieve a particular outcome.

mudra Positions or gestures, usually made with the hands and fingers. In the yoga tradition, *mudras* are said to further stimulate and direct *prana* and offer a point of focus for the mind.

nadi A channel through which energy flows in our bodies. The three central *nadis* are *ida*, *pingala*, and *sushumna*. The *nadis* are said to connect at points of intensity at our chakras.

nadi shodhana Alternate nostril breathing or channel-cleaning breathing.

parasympathetic nervous system One half of the body's autonomic nervous system, responsible for keeping our basic bodily functions working as they should and triggering the body's 'rest and digest' response.

prana Life force or vital energy.

pranayama Techniques for focusing on the breath and regulating vital energy.

sama vritti Equal breathing or box breathing.

simhasana pranayama Lion's breath.

sitali pranayama Cooling breath.

sukhasana Sitting cross-legged.

surya bhedana Sun-piercing breath. A breathing practice that focuses on the right nostril. Practised together with *chandra bhedana,* it forms alternate nostril breathing.

sympathetic nervous system One half of the body's autonomic nervous system, responsible for reacting to danger and triggering the body's 'fight or flight' response.

ujjayi breath Victorious breath or ocean breath.

vagus nerve One of the 12 cranial nerves, the vagus is the longest nerve in the autonomic nervous system, often called the wandering nerve. It is responsible for carrying signals between the brain and the heart, lungs, and digestive tract.

Practice Charts

Here we have included a handy practice chart for your reference, which includes the suggested practices for each day. We have also provided a blank version in case you would like to create your own practice schedule. You can also download copies of these charts at https://library.jkp.com/redeem using the code WLDEQJK.

Week 1	Day 1	Day 2	Day 3	Day 4	Day 5	Day 6	Day 7
	• Breath awareness	• *Sama vritti* (equal breathing): beginner's	• Breath awareness • *Simhasana pranayama* (lion's breath)	• *Ujjayi* breath (victorious breath/ocean breath): beginner's	• Extended exhalation	• *Surya bhedana* (alternate nostril breathing/sun-piercing breath)	• *Chandra bhedana* (alternate nostril breathing/moon-piercing breath)
	⏱ 5 minutes	⏱ 5 minutes	⏱ 5 minutes	⏱ 5 minutes	⏱ 5 minutes	⏱ 5 minutes – practise in the am	⏱ 5 minutes – practise in the pm

Week 2	Day 8	Day 9	Day 10	Day 11	Day 12	Day 13	Day 14
	• Breath awareness • *Sama vritti* (equal breathing): beginner's • *Sitali pranayama* (cooling breath – suggest up to 2 minutes of this practice)	• Breath awareness • *Bhramari pranayama* (bee breath)	• Breath awareness • *Sama vritti* (equal breathing): beginners	• Breath awareness • *Ujjayi* breath (victorious breath/ocean breath)	• Breath awareness • *Simhasana pranayama* (lion's breath)	• Extended exhalation • *Sitali pranayama* (cooling breath)	• Extended exhalation • *Bhramari pranayama* (bee breath)
	⏱ 5–10 minutes	⏱ 5–10 minutes	⏱ 5–10 minutes	⏱ 5–10 minutes	⏱ 5–10 minutes	⏱ 5–10 minutes	⏱ 5–10 minutes

Week 3	Day 15	Day 16	Day 17	Day 18	Day 19	Day 20	Day 21
	• *Sama vritti* (box breathing – advanced)	• *Ujjayi* breath (victorious breath/ocean breath): advanced	• *Nadi shodhana* (alternate nostril breathing): advanced	• Sun breath	• *Dirga pranayama* (three-part yogic breath/jug breath)	• Breath awareness • *Kapalabhati* (skull-shining breath)	• Breath awareness • *Surya bhedana* (alternate nostril breathing/sun-piercing breath)
	⏱ 5 minutes	⏱ 5 minutes	⏱ 5 minutes	⏱ 5 minutes	⏱ 5 minutes	⏱ 5 minutes – practise in the am	⏱ 5–10 minutes – practise in the am

Week 4	Day 22	Day 23	Day 24	Day 25	Day 26	Day 27	Day 28
	• Breath awareness • *Chandra bhedana* (alternate nostril breathing/moon-piercing breath)	• *Sama vritti* (box breathing): advanced • *Ujjayi* breath (victorious breath/ocean breath): advanced	• *Sama vritti* (box breathing): advanced • Sun breath • *Dirga pranayama* (three-part breath/jug breath)	• *Kapalabhati* (skull-shining breath) • *Sama vritti* (box breathing): advanced • *Ujjayi* breath (victorious breath/ocean breath): advanced	• *Sama vritti* (equal breathing): beginner's • *Bhramari pranayama* (bee breath) • *Nadi shodhana* (alternate nostril breathing): advanced • Sun breath	• Freestyle – choose your favourite practices	• Freestyle – choose your favourite practices
	⏱ 10 minutes – practise in the pm	⏱ 10 minutes	⏱ 10–15 minutes	⏱ 10–15 minutes	⏱ 15 minutes	⏱ 15 minutes	⏱ 15 minutes

Week 1	Day 1	Day 2	Day 3	Day 4	Day 5	Day 6	Day 7

Week 2	Day 8	Day 9	Day 10	Day 11	Day 12	Day 13	Day 14

Week 3	Day 15	Day 16	Day 17	Day 18	Day 19	Day 20	Day 21

Week 4	Day 22	Day 23	Day 24	Day 25	Day 26	Day 27	Day 28

References

De Couck, M., Caers, R., Much, L., *et al.* (2019) 'How breathing can help you make better decisions: Two studies on the effects of breathing patterns on heart rate variability and decision-making in business cases.' International Journal of Psychophysiology, 139: 1–9. https://www.sciencedirect.com/science/article/abs/pii/S0167876018303258

Divine, M. (2016, May 4) 'The breathing technique a Navy SEAL uses to stay calm and focused.' TIME. https://time.com/4316151/breathing-technique-navy-seal-calm-focused/

Iyengar, B. K. S. (2001) Light on Yoga. London: Thorsons.

Mosley, M. (2023) Just One Thing: How Simple Changes Can Transform Your Life. London: Short Books.

Nestor, J. (2020) Breath: The New Science of a Lost Art. London: Penguin Life.

Sovik, R. (n.d.) 'Joyous mind: The practice of nadi shodhanam (alternate nostril breathing).' *Yoga International.* https://yogainternational.com/article/view/joyous-mind/

Acknowledgements

The publishers would like to thank Katie Forsythe, Sarah Hamlin, Masooma Malik, Claire Wilson, Sandra Nimako-Boatey, Katelynn Bartleson, Adam Peacock, Carys Homer, Winsey Samuels, Nicola Powling, Aggie Stewart, Jenny Edwards, Carole McMurray, Mark Scott, Emily Short, Olivia Bromage, David Corey, Stephanie DeMuzio, Julia Zullo, Claire Shewbridge, and Rosamund Bird.

About the Publishers

Singing Dragon publishes authoritative books on yoga and yoga therapy, Chinese medicine, nutrition and lifestyle medicine, aromatherapy, and more, for health, wellbeing, and professional and personal development. Singing Dragon was founded in 2006 and is an imprint of Jessica Kingsley Publishers.

In 2022 Singing Dragon acquired Handspring Publishing, recognised as the leading publisher in the fields of manual therapies and movement.

www.singingdragon.com